Table of Contents

Preface and Dedication - I've been there
2

Copyright and Disclaimer Information
4

Where do You Start?
6

Have to Feed The Abs - The Right Way
12

The Part You'll "Get Around To" (Read It Now, Not Later)
19

Let's Talk About Your Ab Training Plan
26

The Wonderful World of Isometrics
33

How to Get Six Pack Abs with a Brown Paper Bag
37

How To Get Six Pack Abs With A Pen and Paper!
39

How to Get Six Pack Abs Starting With the Basics
42

We Need Hydration, ever Consider Alkaline Water?
45

Do You Start Off With Stress?
47

It's Not The End
50

Preface and Dedication - I've been there

In life there's a great deal of importance placed on the "why's" and "how's". Court cases and scientific breakthroughs are dependent upon answering these questions. History relies on the answer to "why" and "how" to go from a folk lore to a fact.

In our personal lives, when we know how something works we stand an advantage. The advantage is that we are able to see a broader spectrum of things. It allows you to piece a variety of complex components together. It also allows you to full grasp an idea for the idea and not just see a superficial aspect.

Exercise is no different; every movement has reasoning behind it. Any form of exercise from the simplest stretch to a complex multi-planular has upwards of thousand of working components that need to be appreciated so they are not ignored. Ignoring the slightest muscle incorporation, or metabolism working, could mean devastation to your workout routine or weight loss plan. With that being said, it makes sense to understand the core workings of your six pack and therefore leads to the introduction of this content investigation of how to get, and how to keep your six pack.

You Made This Possible

Mom, you never gave up on me and your dedication made me realize I can help other people, this book is for you. You not only taught me to figure out the "what" of life but the importance of respecting and knowing the "why" of the "what" I find.

Dad, you've gone through up's and down's however you show extreme determination in achieving your personal goals on a master type of level. I cannot say I commend you as that would be a blatant understatement.

Brie, Owie, and James, you three are my world, I love you three equally and want you to continue understanding why. I want you three to follow the principals I set in this book and have as long and happy life with many successes as you each allow yourselves. I could not ask for more enjoyable and inspirational children than you.

Sammi and Russ, you've each helped me through my personal lows and push me to strive for my potential in its highest form. You encourage me to find a way to help the masses and give back, which is why I put my heart into this book. Sammi I can't wait until we are husband and wife, hopefully this is how I can tell the world.

My Lord Jesus Christ - I truly believe I can do all things through You who strengthens me.

Copyright and Disclaimer Information

I'll make this fast and easy, if you reuse any of my work in this book you agree to pay me 5,000 times the highest purchase price as a resale based product and agree to cover any legal fees and fees directly or indirectly related to any legal proceedings.

This book is based on my thoughts and my own personal research. They should be used for informational and educational purposes only. As with any decision in life the responsibility is yours to research and seek medical advice before trying anything. You agree to hold me harmless in any result from you attempting to put into action any of the ideas laid out in this book. It is your responsibility to consult with your doctor.

I'll paraphrase this, This book is a collection of my thoughts, findings, and experiences as a personal trainer and someone who studies health related topics. I'll never claim my medical advice will work better than a doctor's, nor can I tell if you are doing an exercise properly. It's up to you to seek out a doctor and trainer and that is not a bad idea!

Pay Attention to the teachings in this book. Occasionally I will recommend a product. Those products are completely optional and are not needed for the principals in this book to work. Again you need to read the Medical disclaimer. Additionally, I may receive compensation if you decide to purchase the product. I have no business relationship with any product or parties recommended in this book, I am solely receiving a commission if you purchase them – I have gone through them myself however, and have no issue putting my name behind them!

Now that my butt is covered let's get into this!

Where do You Start?

Let Six Pack Abs Strike Your Body!

Six pack abs are probably one of the hottest year round commodities in the United States, and are also becoming one world wide as countries begin to develop more. For many, who do not research properly on how to attain them, they are also a pipe dream. Some people work out feverishly trying to attain those highly desired abs, and are left disappointed as they don't make any notable progress at all!

So what do you need to focus on and use as a starting point to get those coveted six pack abs? You're in luck as I'll be sharing that with you. Your quest will require an understanding and implementation of a proper diet (yes there's a difference between a good and bad diet), regular exercise (different types), one heck of a positive mindset (I will cover why in a bit), and motivation!

It Takes Some Exercise To Get Abs For Showing!

Exercise, although it is not the only way (and should not be seen as the only way), is the traditional first step when thinking about how getting a core that will leave other envious. Which body part do we exercise? Mainstream acceptance suggests that to get six pack abs you just do crunches, right? Wrong!

Truth be, told there are actually four parts to the core, and each needs to get some exercise attention paid to them. With that being said, which muscles make up the famous and picturesque six pack abs we see in magazines and movies, well pretty much anywhere they can be advertised?

Let's start from the inside out, first up are the **transverse abdominus**. These are the inner abdominal muscles in your six pack abs. The transverse abdominus has two extremely important jobs and neither has to do with vanity reasons. They work as a fortress does to protect a castle, or a desert outpost, however in regards to your body they protect most of the organs in your trunk. Your trunk is pretty much your entire midsection. This leaves us with the second important task your transverse abdominus handle, they work to stabilize your trunk and keep a balance in you.

Do you remember your mother or father telling you to stand up straight and "suck it in"? They are referring to indirectly the second job of your transverse abdominus.

Who's up next in our six pack ab musculature quartet? That would be your **rectus abdominus**! What does the rectus abdominus do? Well, the rectus abdominus is not just a funny name (but it certainly sounds like one), it also give off that nice looking six pack appearance! The rectus abdominus does not just make your six pack abs look pretty; they also dictate the tilt of your pelvis as well as improve the mechanics of the erector spinae. So you can pretty much compare your rectus abdominus to the super hot girl who had some killer brains as well!

We touched on the transverse and rectus abdominus, so that leaves two more muscle groups in what makes our six pack work properly and show. We also have a double take on the oblique area! Let me explain, your six pack abs have two other important players - the **internal obliques** as well as **external obliques**, but what do they do for your six pack abs? Well, the internal obliques are pretty cool as they are the inside man (my shot at humor). On a serious note they actually aid in allowing your midsection to twist properly.

For example, I am a huge baseball fan and if a hitter's mechanics are off and he takes a swing from the right side, there's a possibility with other muscles groups over compensating his right internal oblique muscles could be hurt.

So before we touch on the last **muscle group,** are you starting to gain a respect for six pack abs as more like an important tool than just a regular sexy set of six pack abs with no significance? We covered three of the important players of your six pack abs, so who is the last muscle set? If you were paying attention (if not, shame shame!), it is the exterior obliques! How could we have strong six pack abs that include the interior obliques but neglect the exterior obliques? The external obliques act as the outside walls protecting the center of a fortress, but yours move. Okay, that was a bad example. When you are turning, they stabilize your core. When that same hitter is swinging (in the internal obliques example) from the left side, the right obliques are being put to use. Make sense?

Eat For Abs!

Now that we have the four heavy hitters of our six pack abs we need to know what to feed them. A strong site I highly recommend is Diabetic Diet Resources, and although not directly tied into six pack abs that site does hit on some hot food ideas, tips, snack tricks and a bunch more. For six pack abs we should consider putting the ice cream cone back inside the freezer. Take that ice cream cone out of the freezer again actually; you will need it for "ransom" on your journey to six pack abs. I am not saying you will get six pack abs via an ice cream truck, however having a "cheat" every once in a while keeps you on track. It also allows you to eat those bumps in the road toward six pack abs.

Six pack abs are a sign of a healthy body, don't you agree? In order to get six pack abs you need to have minimal fat around your transverse and rectus abdominus as well as your interior and exterior obliques (remember the previous paragraphs? They highlight the mandatory body parts behind six pack abs and won't cut through fat on their own!). This means the boring six pack abs diet. Lean steak, fish, steamed or grilled veggies and fruit, sounds gut wrenching right? I did not think so either!

While you WILL need some fat in your diet (actually, the fish mentioned would provide some very healthy **omega 3**'s) to achieve six pack abs it can be tasty! Coconut oil is my personal favorite fat.
Six pack abs can come naturally if you treat them and nourish them properly. That being said you should highly consider naturally nurturing your six pack abs with **whole foods** and try as much as you can to stay away from the processed stuff.

I am not by any stretch saying to outlaw it from your diet (unless you can!) however the whole foods are easier for your body to break down and normally do not have any of their vitamin, mineral, and **amino acid** densities broken down. It's also easy to substitute these items! Whole grains and whole wheat unbleached flour make feeding your six pack abs ready body even easier!

It's All In Your Head

Any diet or exercise regimen is going to be tough to follow at first. Actually any journey or trip you have never taken or have not embarked on in some time will be a challenge at first. There's a good reason for this, and understanding it will help you on your journey. As humans we become comfortable with routine. If you've been non-active and eat fast food for ages transforming your life is going to be more difficult. You are comfortable in your ways.

There are going to be days when you lose track of time and can't get that workout in. There'll be days when you forget the salad you or your spouse made for work and you'll have to stop and grab something as you need food to function. That's OK just don't let those very slight and temporary slip ups dictate your transformation process.

The road to six pack abs that you can wash your clothes on near a river's edge (major exaggeration) is no less difficult. In fact, when you hit a plateau you may say "I'd rather drink a six pack instead of get six pack abs instead" you may literally throw in the towel.

If you are reading this I assume you are at least 10 or can understand some words, so here's a question unrelated at first to your six pack abs journey, have you ever had a bad day? After that initial bad day, had your next day normally taken a turn for the better? This is no different. I have a very good life however, I have had really bad days but I do not let them dictate my future. Rarely will a day in time create the rest of your life.

Your mindset is going to play a pivotal role in literally all aspects of your life. Actually, what you feed your brain can effect what you are able to put out. Telling yourself that six pack abs are never going to be found as your midsection is allowing yourself to be told (you hear your own words) that you will never get six pack abs. However, being able to vividly picture yourself with six pack abs will make the end goal of your six pack abs journey so much more possible it is ridiculous! You need something at the end of the road to motivate yourself to get there.

Motivate Yourself

Why do you want to increase your core strength and transform your life? What will taking action with the concepts and ideas in this book do for you? Do yourself a favor and write down why you are doing this. Picture what you want to look like, what you want to feel like. Picture yourself living a full life.

An easy way to get you on track doing this is to go to a dollar store and buy a sticky note or something. Write down why you are doing this and stick it on the fridge, on top of the TV. Place it in your "bad spots" that cause you to stray from your goals and life objectives. Ask yourself if you're exercising during commercials, ask yourself if you can use some olive oil and herbs and stick that one on your refrigerator.

These seemingly simple tips can help you stay on path. How do I know? They worked for me, and they've worked for numerous personal training clients of mine. The tests proved to work, and if you let them they will work for you as well!

Have to Feed The Abs - The Right Way

When thinking about a long-term and sustainable diet on your six pack quest, you need to realize it is a way of life. Think about it, eating healthy *is* a way of life. Going against what you are striving to do will lead to three things, a **sedentary lifestyle, obesity**, and major health complications that stem from a poor **lifestyle**. Look at the USA today, TV and tasks that require little to no movement are the norm. **Gluttonous** days, such as Thanksgiving, have turned into a typical Sunday activity after church (isn't our body our Lord's temple anyway?). There's no denying food has become a lifestyle.

Being said, if you are new to diets or dieting, you can look at your food choices one of two ways, what your six pack abs diet can contain or what you six pack abs diet cannot contain. From experience as a personal trainer and life coach, I can tell you that the latter thought process will make your dieting extremely difficult. Most humans hate being told no.

Looking at what you cannot eat is a very, very poor and negative way to view your dieting approach. Train yourself to get excited and interested with what you can eat. As I've mentioned you are now on a quest or journey, you are your own trail blazer or pioneer. Take advantage of the fact you are going to be going to new food taste destinations you have never been (remember, "Where Do You Start" places importance in mindset - psych yourself up). So let's look at a few things we want to eat which we'll cover along with some ideas!

You want to have a mixture of simple carbohydrates as well as complex carbohydrates. You want healthy and good for you fats and you want lean protein in your diet. Let us stay with a whole food mentality and stay away from the processed foods.

Foods Do Not Like Processing!

Processed foods are everywhere due to their ease which plays along lovely in our instant gratification based society. It is also easy to realize these foods can make you pay a steep price and sabotage any progress made in your six pack abs diet. What types of foods are in your current diet could be processed? Take a peak in your cupboard and refrigerator. Take a peek at the ingredient list, if you have say a whole grain tortilla and the first ingredient isn't a whole grain, there's an issue. If you feel the need to break open a chemistry book to see what you're eating, you may not want to digest it - just saying.

In fact, if you look at any Facebook nutrition page there's a chance you will see infographics highlighting common processing agents. In fact, you can even do a simple search engine query and probably find those same foods linked to increases in genetic manipulation, cancer, and many other nasty things. Go and take a search or two. I'll apologize ahead of time if you feel the need to put this book down and go food shopping.

Processing isn't just detrimental and wasteful due to the chemical agents placed in them. There is added salt for meat based products to extend shelf life, which isn't too good for your blood pressure. Aside from that, the nutrients completely disappear. Let's take a peek at rice for example, shall we?

When rice is bleached, a ton of the nutrient density goes with the coloring making white rice (in my opinion as a six pack abs diet fan) a glorified starch. I will still use white rice once in a great while, however only for a super duper quick fix if I am out too long with the kids on a walk or something along those lines. The six pack abs diet also does not care that much for flour. Scratch that, the six pack abs diet hates white flour and why not? Why would you eat something with no nutritional value?

Instead of using flour, what I did was actually toy around with steel cut or Irish oatmeal. It gives food a different taste, and with some seasoning, it can give a great and wholesome effect, once you adjust to the new texture (sorry, no getting around that one). In addition, it is oatmeal, can you think of something with good carbs and some protein for breakfast that fills you up more? I will throw it on chicken any day of the week with some rosemary and Tabasco.

Add Some Fats (the Right Ones) and See A Six Pack

Fats are no different as they can be mass-produced and human created easily. Your new diet wants you to have some fats in your food consumption, and in fact encourages it, but what types? Take a look at the type of fats we have available to us. We have saturated fats, trans fats, monounsaturated, and polyunsaturated fats. Can you guess which ones fit into the six pack abs diet? Monounsaturated and polyunsaturated are good fats, which help your body, live – they use them (as well as carbohydrates) for energy!

Many fad diets boast the ability to use protein for energy – not the world's best idea. Monounsaturated and polyunsaturated fats can be found in foods ranging from oil to nuts (olive oil, omega 3's, corn oil, etc.).

The easiest way to see if you are about to pound some good fats or bad fats at the dinner table is literally how the uncooked fat looks. Monounsaturated and polyunsaturated fats are liquid in form (i.e. olive oil) where the bad fats are solid at room temperature (think margarine and butter or animal lard). Experiment with healthy fats, or a more liquid fat and your dieting results will thank you down the road (not to mention your heart and other vital organs)!

Don't Skip on Carbs, Just Eat the Right Ones!

Carbohydrates work the same way as fats, although the bad carbohydrate isn't as bad as the bad fats (say that 10 times fast). Complex carbohydrates feed your body a long released carbohydrate. Simple carbohydrates are shorter in length and turn into unused energy (fat) faster than the complex counterparts. Although bad fats can cause heart disease and could be grounds for a bypass down the road, simple carbohydrates make you more prone to diabetes if, like almost anything else, you abuse them. Complex carbohydrates also help you feel satisfied longer (candy bar full of sugar [simple] compared to oatmeal [complex]).

My initial six pack abs diet was extremely similar to the one I'll be covering for an example shortly. Any six pack abs diet needs limited amounts of the bad fats and bad carbohydrates. Actually here is what simple carbohydrates can do to your six pack abs diet – they can give you potbelly syndrome, make you hate your six pack abs diet because your results will start slipping, and leave you feeling sluggish. A six pack abs diet, when eaten healthy, will make your diet a pot belly's worst enemy!

What About A Bit 'O Protein?

As I mentioned before, protein is a crucial element in the six pack abs diet, but the right kind. Someone on a diet will come across a couple different kinds of proteins. They are whey, isolate, casein, and one so crappy I will not mention it. Those are not suppose to be part of your six pack abs diet as I am a firm believer that a whole food diet will give you health nutrients and with some spices will make your six pack abs diet a success!

But after a hard workout, a shake may not be that bad. Unless you're like me and pack a hummus and broccoli container for your post workout snack.

Before I mentioned you want all three energy sources (carbs, fat, and protein) as part of your six pack abs diet and that you shouldn't allow your six pack abs diet to use protein as an energy source. Why? Your body uses protein for probably a million or so biological functions.

Most importantly, while you are exercising as part of your new health journey you will (naturally – don't worry) rip muscles. That is why many love the idea of a full glass of milk within a half hour of ending your workout. Not to rip muscles, however between them and amino acids you start a repair process which kicks into over drive when you're sleeping.

So What's the Plate Going to Look Like?

So what is the plate setup I mentioned your six pack abs diet plate should resemble? I do one-half complex carbohydrates one quarter simple carbohydrate or as I call them starchy carb, and one quarter protein.

I know you read up on the topic and are wondering "why does only one quarter of my six pack abs diet plate have protein?". The answer to that is how often does a food only contain fat, only contain protein, or only contain a carbohydrate? It normally does not work that way unless the topic of conversation is lard.

In fact, beans could wind up on your plate and not only are they a carbohydrate full of good fiber but also contain protein! As does something like tuna fish or salmon which actually does not count as they are meat and take up a quarter of your plate anyway. Regardless, eating a well rounded healthy whole food diet will not only increase the results of your six pack abs diet but also your life.

Your new diet does not have to be mundane. In fact, this new lifestyle you are getting into will only be mundane and tough to stick with if you are too lazy to read labels or fear playing around with seasoning.

 In case you're leery of playing with spices, here's a tip: spicy foods can heat your body up through their thermogenic properties meaning weight loss is going to come even easier! Aside from that, you can also clear your sinuses by eating spicy foods!

Two big questions only you can answer:

How are you going to start your six pack abs diet? (Actually, I told you how,)

WHEN are you going to start your six pack abs diet?

The Part You'll "Get Around To"
(Read It Now, Not Later)

Diet does, did, and will play a huge role in your quest for a rock hard six pack - you're in control of the fat that gets stored over your abs. If you don't have any abs to show off because you don't work them out, would you say your core is healthy?

You have to do more than consider exercise if you want healthy, popping, and toned core muscles - you have to do the exercise. That is only if you want your results to show. I haven't seen so much debate on one topic as I have with six pack ab exercises! Some will tell you it is all about the intensity, or this workout plan or only this exercise to end your routine. I say blah to it all and will give you an analogy for why I say that.

Roy Halladay is probably the best pitcher our era has/will see. He performs consistently at champion caliber. He adds a new pitch every once in a while and what do you think he does with the others? He keeps training his repertoire regularly, not just that one pitch. Would it make sense to only focus on one aspect of core strength training than? Do what a pitcher does, focus on one solid pitch and confuse the batter by adding new pitches, or in your case exercises.

Has it been a while?

If it has been a while or if you are just starting your first six pack ab routine, do you think it would be wise to start doing what you see trained and ripped people in the gym doing? Actually, I digress momentarily; there is a benefit to that. It's a perfect way to set goals for where your six pack ab exercises will lead to. Now I'm back on track, initially you will hurt yourself or have a greatly increased risk of injury to yourself if you're trying to keep up with a professional or very seasoned and regular body builder. There are a lot of reasons for this; however I think that two of those reasons are very preventable.

The first issue I have run into quite often as a personal trainer is walking to your ab exercises mat with the "all exercises are the same, you work out" attitude. All exercises are not a "one size fits all" idea, in fact they all vary on levels ranging from beginner to advanced and six pack ab exercises are no different. On the same token, don't forget your abs have 4 different muscles that make them up.

Another common issue with people walking into training is trying to do an advanced workout with untrained abs and poor form. Six pack ab exercises are not only made to strengthen and exploit the fruits of your labor, however also to stabilize your core!

Poor form during six pack ab exercises can slow the progress you are aiming for. In fact, some six pack ab exercises work more muscle groups than most other exercises. In fact, I considered major classes during my training days ab exercises, the inclined bench press, squats and properly done push ups. If you have poor form in any of those, including six pack ab exercises, you can mess up the form and posture of other muscle groups involved.

The major classes I mentioned including six pack ab exercises involve multiple muscle groups. Work on your form prior to jumping into heavy and innovated exercises along those lines especially six pack ab exercises.

Confusion is in the curriculum!

We already covered which muscle groups are in your trunk and each of those needs to be worked! They do not need to be the same mundane sit-up you learned in Phys. Ed during middle school. However, you do need to add some confusing and challenge to them.

Confusing your muscles with new six pack ab exercises could also help you burn more of that fat wall blocking your six pack! This type of six pack ab exercises are normally done when you feel your six pack ab exercises need a more intermediate or advanced level of training.

The most important aspect, in my opinion, of a six pack ab exercises routine is not what you do with you stomach, but rather your hand. Your mind is real important when it comes to six pack ab exercises also actually. Do you know which exercise I am referring to? If you guessed will power, you are half wrong. Will power is important, but I will cover will power later on, what does will power have to do with your hand anyway?. It is your journal that you jot stuff down in! This little guy helps you do tons of things from planning to analyzing. You can check out your progress or regression from results (covered down the road, very important topic!).

Six pack ab exercises come in all shapes and forms. Most six pack ab exercises involve a crunch-motion of some type, however some six pack ab exercises involve your entire trunk. The six pack ab exercises that target and activate the muscles in your entire core are normally advanced (past intermediate). My favorite six pack ab exercises are the bicycle crunch as well as the rapidly becoming popular kneeling wood chopper.

Those two six pack ab exercises will have your stomach screaming for mercy. To make those two six pack ab exercises a little more difficult I will even attach a resistance band to something and crunch that way!

Earlier I mentioned training as part of your six pack ab exercises, as with any other muscle group you need to rest your abs, especially if you are just starting off. A way of relating what happens if you practice day in and day out your six pack ab exercises is with a rubber band. A rubber band works fine at room temperature, however what happens to the band if it gets used on a regular and ongoing basis? Eventually the rubber band will snap or be so loose it's pointless to use. Your abs after six pack ab exercises are no different and also need a break.

Although it is not the only way to get six pack abs, you need to implement a six pack abs workout to get results. Planning, accountability, determination, diet, and so many other items are needed, however they do not make up for a six pack abs workout.

Your workout doesn't know when to stop, but you do!

Another important fact you need to grasp is that you need to know your limitations. I have not dedicated an entire session strictly to a six pack abs workout in a while. I decided recently I was just going to focus on my abdominals and get back into a six pack abs workout. I tell clients regularly that they should take baby steps when getting back into an exercise program.

When I went to do my own six pack abs workout I should have taken my own advice. I was doing some advanced six pack abs exercises and found at around 15 reps my form was becoming shaky. I also noticed I had to take more breaks at a higher frequency than normal.

Another "obvious" piece of advice for your six pack abs workout is to take account of your results and failures. This will help you in a few ways with your six pack abs workout sessions. First, reviewing it after a break will give you an idea of what you did during the recent exercises.

Another way writing down what you do during your workouts is that when you find yourself stuck in a non-productive funk or plateau you can see where your reps are sky rocketing and potentially add a more advanced variation to that specific six pack abs exercise. Actually, when you find yourself looking for a change, going over your track record may show you an area you have been progressing in regularly and you could swap an exercise or two in.

Another benefit of writing down the results from your six pack abs workout is when you feel like you want to throw in the towel and quit. Sometimes, actually closer to normally, we never realize our true production until we can "take 5" and see just how far we have come.

Six pack workouts aren't what they use to be!

The six pack abs workout has come quite a way from where the concept started. I remember as a youth that if we wanted to get six pack abs we were told to knock out as many crunches as we could handle. Not only is this counter-productive, what about the rest of your core? I guess if you were to purposely trigger and brace your entire core that you may be able to get by although I would imagine your six pack abs workout would get very boring.

What happens when something gets boring, six pack abs workout or attending church when you have a choice? You stop doing it! So what sort of spice can we add to our six pack abs workout to make the recipe "not as bland"? Well let's hit the muscles we should make sure our six pack abs workout targets, keep reading.

Do you remember on another page where I discussed what makes up a healthy set of six pack abs? I'll repeat it, not word for word but close with a new addition! Look at your six pack abs for a second, do you know what makes them a six pack? There is more than one muscle hiding in there.

Earlier in this book, I threw out words where you may have thought I was speaking another language. If you want some solid six pack abs workouts than you need to target your core or trunk muscles. These are your internal and external obliques as well as your transverse and rectus abdominis.

Now it's time to throw an additional muscle group into your six pack abs workout! That would be none other than your lower back. That sounds weird doesn't it? What does your lower back have to do with getting six pack abs? A lot actually, let's start with the obvious fact first. Where on your body is your lower back? Now tell me where your six pack is, can you see what I'm getting at? What happens when you have lower back pain or poor posture? You bend forward, after successful six pack abs workout sessions this could make it appear you have 6 rolls instead of perfectly formed rocks forming the six pack we all want!

Throw some of these into your workout

I have mentioned a six pack abs workout a couple times so far, but haven't given any specific workouts. The other paragraphs cover more of an information approach, specifically information you should know prior to the working out. Let us go over some exercises you can add to any six pack abs workout session. I would perform the exercises I mention below before your regular workout. As always, and this cannot be stressed enough, you absolutely have to discuss any exercise or diet program with a doctor.

One exercise I do to strengthen my lower back is the "Super Man". I start by laying on my stomach with my hands shoulder stretched in front off my body as if I am reaching for something. I then raise my extended legs and arms while slightly bringing my shoulders and head off the ground and go back to the starting position. That makes one "rep" and I typically perform 5 "reps". I initially raise myself 3 inches off the ground and with each rep I increase the distance I raise myself off the ground by an additional 3 inches. I hold each rep for 10 seconds.

How about another exercise for your six pack abs workout? This one is actually easier than most and triggers your "hidden" ab muscles. For this exercise you want to grab a roll of tape or a CD case. Next you lay on your back with your knees at a 45 degree angle, looking similar to your lower leg and thigh making the sides of a triangle. Next, place the CD case or roll of tape on your belly button and place your palms on the floor. Now, take a deep breath and as you exhale contract your abs. Keep the contraction and begin lowering the item on your belly button toward your spin. Keeping the contraction, you want to take another deep breath and as you exhale contract your abs a little more and lower the item a bit closer to your spine.

Although these items are very basic, they are important additions to your six pack abs workout. In fact, regardless if it a chest workout or a six pack abs workout you can only progress when you can add to flawlessly executed fundamentals. I feel adding these workouts to your six pack abs workout should provide noticeable stability and core strength results.

Let's Talk About Your Ab Training Plan

An overlooked concept that has been making the rounds again, HIIT Training, might just be the answer to your hunt for a new and different **six pack workout**. HIIT stands for High Intensity Interval Training, and involves doing specific periods of high intensity, high cardio training coupled with lower levels of cardio training.

This system is different from your run-of-the-mill interval training in that the periods of high intensity are higher and the periods of rest are shorter than in regular interval training. It is entirely possible to complete an entire workout in 10 to 15 minutes using HIIT.

This type of workout is perfect for people who are looking to supercharge their six pack workout routine, get off a training or weight loss plateau, or anyone who is simply bored with what they are doing.

Background of HIIT: Fartlek Inspired

No, it's not an impolite word. It simply means 'speed play' in Swedish. The first early examples of HIIT were developed in the mid 1930's by a running coach named Gosta Holmér. He was tired of seeing his cross country teams get beat all of the time, so he developed Fartlek as a way to increase their speed and endurance. His system measured the cardiac output of his athletes as they completed sprints.

He soon found that not only did Fartlek improve their overall aerobic capacity; it greatly improved their speed and long-term endurance. The beauty of his system is that over the decades it has proven to be highly adaptable to all types of sports, and it is similar to the quick bursts of activity that occur in sports like basketball, soccer, and football. A version of it is also currently used in Quantico Va. to train officer candidates for the Marine Corps.

The Science behind HIIT

As noted by S. Boucher (University of New South Whales, School of Medical Sciences) there have been numerous medical studies that seem to indicate that true HIIT training can result not only in a high degree of fat loss, but also improvements in aerobic and anaerobic fitness, and a significant decrease in insulin resistance, which is terrific news for anyone with diabetes.

The effects on people with diabetes and people that are severely obese have shown promise in assisting them to normalize blood glucose levels and lose weight in an effective manner. Studies that measured insulin response to HIIT show an increase of up to 58% sensitivity to insulin. This is compared to a response rate of about 33% in non-diabetic test subjects. Some studies have shown that this benefit can last as long as three days, although for most people it lasted 3-24 hours. Most diabetics will take any positive.

HIIT activates what are known as fast twitch muscle fibers. These are the muscle fibers that gave us the natural ability to run away from danger back at the beginning of the human race. These fibers use more energy to fire and recover, making it possible to lose more weight compared to longer interval training (jogging at a slower pace on a treadmill for 20 minutes).

HIIT sends the body into an anabolic working state that is similar to weight training, but that involved the entire body. An awesome after-effect of a HIIT training session is see in increased fat burning capacity for several hours after your training session. This composes an additive that could help create a near perfect six pack workout routine.

Why HIIT It for a Six Pack Workout

Not sold on the information so far? Let's keep digging in! One of the many advantages of high intensity interval training (HIIT) is that is takes a very short amount of time to complete a workout as mentioned above. Completing a HIIT workout in about 10 minutes can easily be both expected and reasonable, considering the level of physical activity. True HIIT training involves working to as close to 100% of your capacity as possible for specifically timed spurts.

If, for example you decide to use a treadmill or stationary bike, you would run as fast as possible for 10 seconds, and then lower your intensity to a mid-level jog for 20 seconds. You would repeat this cycle for 4-6 sets in a 10 (starting off) to 15 (when you build up your stamina a bit) minute workout session.

The true key to this type of six pack workout is intensity; it really is a critical component in having a successful HIIT routine. It will cause extreme discomfort to be at this level of training-Most people use what's called the Borg Scale of Perceived Exertion. This scale is a self measure tool that works on how you feel while doing the exercise. It generally goes from 1-10, with 1 being the lowest level of exertion and 10 being "I feel like I'm dying" level.

The hard core, high intensity level training sends your muscles into an anaerobic state requiring your entire body to work to complete the workout. This leads to additional fat burn that extends to periods long after the initial workout.

When Not to HIIT It

This high level high intensity can also be one of the drawbacks to doing a HIIT workout. This type of training can be intensely uncomfortable. If you have any underlying medical conditions, this workout should only be attempted if you've checked with and gotten the okay from your healthcare provider.

If you are severely obese or have not worked out in awhile, you will need to start at a slower pace or fewer sets initially. To add another portion to this equation, I'd really consider having someone watching you while doing this and be in some contact with your doctor to monitor results.

One of the muscles that will be responding to this type of workout is your heart. If it has taken a beating through exertion due to cholesterol or other potential components, the reason toward my recommendation should make sense.

Anyone with cardiac problems should probably not attempt it at all to be on the safe side. If you truly desire it (dreams are what make life complete – that is when we achieve them) you should do so under medical guidance ads well as observance.

This workout will place a great amount of stress on your cardio-vascular system. Your heartbeat could go as high as 170 during the intense phase and will not drop by much until after the session is complete. You will have difficulty breathing as well, even if you are in reasonably good shape.

Being said, if you are asthmatic or have pulmonary concerns you may want to take the same advice as I recommended above.

How about we try a fast (no pun intended) HIIT routine?!

Step 1

For the standard HIIT six pack workout you should warm up for about 3 minutes at about a level 2 or 3 intensity. You'll be at a pace that you could maintain long term. Along with the walking warm-up you will want to do some light stretching for your legs to prevent hurting yourself.

Step 2
For the actual exercise phase, you will increase the treadmill to as fast as you can go, pretty much an all out run. This will jolt your body's flight or fight response and will result in the increases in heartbeat and breathing mentioned earlier. After 10 seconds of all out running, slow to a moderate or brisk paced walk or slow jog for 20 seconds.

Repeat these steps 6-8 times. It may seem easy, but be warned. You will find that it will get increasingly more difficult to complete each set as you go. This is the way it's supposed to be. You may find that completing even a few of these is too intense, do as many as you can safely. Try to work up to a total of 8 sets of this for the entire workout.

After you have achieved this HIIT level (8 sets), you can work on increasing the amount of time spent in the all out run phase. Gradually increase your run phase to 15 seconds, with a 45 second 'rest' in between where you are doing your moderate to brisk walk/jog. Note that the recovery time is double the workout time. This is important as you increase or decrease times on your own. We aiming to have our HIIT training equal a 1:2 ratio of effort to rest.

If you want my opinion, HIIT should not be done more than every other day. The reasoning behind this is that you will not receive greater benefits by doing more. In fact you open yourself up to over-training and injuries if you don't allow your body to rest in between HIIT days.

How About Tabata Training? Tabata Whata?

Tabata training is virtually identical to HIIT in that it is very high intensity cardio training. However, more recent developments with Tabata allow you to incorporate high intensity *strength* exercises as well! These exercises include some six pack workout favorites including squats, pushups and lunges. Tabata can also easily be combined with kettle bell or balance ball training.

Some people will decide at this point to go on to do their regular training, this is a good time to add in some resistance or weight exercises from your six pack workout to your routine as your body is primed for maximum energy expenditures.

There are many different programs out there that offer all sorts of complicated routines for doing HIIT. There are even a few people selling specific and very expensive machines for these types of workouts. I really don't think they're needed. Each might have their advantages, I believe that for a six pack workout the simple approach is the best.

At its stripped down best, HIIT is all about maximizing your workout in an efficient manner to get good results. You can do this work out with a treadmill, a stationary bike, a regular bike, or my favorite which is a stopwatch and my own two feet.

There are many ways to incorporate HIIT into your six pack workout, and you may want to consider making it a regular part of your workout!

The Wonderful World of Isometrics

Isometric exercises are just another way to get six pack abs or those dreamy six pack abs. When working toward getting your abs, there are a couple of different forms of exercise you can use and picking which one works the best can be difficult.

The reason that they differ are that they have main underlying principals. For example, aerobic exercise is geared toward endurance where anaerobic exercises are aimed toward increasing your strength. Those are not the only options; in fact for beginners just starting beginning their journey toward six pack abs, I normally recommend *isometric exercises* for six pack abs to start with. Even better, isometric exercises are different too!

The dynamics of isometric exercise is vastly different to those with the previously mentioned anaerobic or aerobic exercises. Instead of seeing results at the full range of motion with a bicep curl or triceps extension, the isometric exercises are more joint-centric. This means they provide most of the results in single solitary area, being the area you are exercising.

Isometric exercises are essentially geared toward that one specific area for a reason. It could be the beginning of a strength training program, or someone going through physical therapy, regardless there is one focal point toward where the focus of the isometric exercises point, for example to the musculature around the joint or knee. Other areas will also be worked and receive some exercise benefits, however they will receive far less than the traditionally dynamic aerobic or anaerobic exercises.

Dynamic exercises trump isometric exercises, especially when considering the abdominal or torso area when you take twitch force of a muscle into consideration. On the other hand, there is no better form of exercise than isometric exercises at enforcing muscle growth or development at the joint angle.

When you have become experienced with isometric exercises you will also find another hidden benefit provided by isometric exercises which is the potential for increased flexibility.

The way you could increase your flexibility through isometric exercise is similar to how you can build a better baseball team during the off season. When completing isometric exercises contractions, your body needs to recruit other muscle fibers that are normally neglected with the traditional dynamic exercises.

How safe are isometric exercises for six pack abs?

Consider weight lifting for a good example of a safety comparison. A better example would be competitively when you are pushing to use heavier weights, exercise is prevalent. This is the biggest reason there are so many safety concerns and even the unwritten requirement of having "spotters" while you are lifting weight.

Isometric exercises on the other hand hold little danger; however, they are not completely out of the dark when it comes to potential safety or danger issues.

The most common form of injury you will find in isometric exercises is the immediate effect on the cardiovascular system. When you are completing an isometric hold, your blood pressure will rise tremendously. If you are not carefully monitoring your breathing or you perform an isometric hold too long, it is not uncommon to become the victim of fainting or even finding yourself having a stroke. When actively personal training, I have found the most common occurrence came with a poor breathing pattern.

Compared to the dynamic exercises this may seem extreme (stole and fainting), although it was only mentioned to show the danger potential. Regardless, there is far greater danger and a much more increased chance of finding injury during the dynamic exercises. The reason for this is a loss of stability at various points of the exercises range of motion.

Other dangerous areas of dynamic exercise are the changing of weight distribution. These potential dangers can lead to a range of injuries ranging from muscle tears, joint damage and in theory even crushing your windpipe if you drop the barbell during a bench press.

Isometric Exercises Help You Keep Your Workout Routine Fair

It's easier not to "cheat" with isometric exercises than it is with other exercises, such as anaerobic. Another area where isometric exercises may prove to be more beneficial are through the lack of cheating motions when you are lifting weights and nearing exhaustion.

Have you ever been to a gym and seen someone working out and rocking so much you are surprised they are not losing their balance? This shows a complete loss of form, which is crucial to receiving maximum benefits of an exercise. Not only can this cause injury, it can also cause the muscle groups to develop unevenly.

This can lead to an increased risk of injury, or cause a poor attitude due to a lack of results.

When you are doing isometric holds, you will find down the road that they do not place the typical demands on form or balance that dynamic exercises do. Another benefit of this is that you cannot compensate for a weaker muscle as the stress is distributed evenly. What that leads to is a better well-rounded development of the joints used in the hold and a safer growth of musculature.

Although you will not receive the bulk you will during a bench press or a supported crunch (a crunch with added weight), the isometric should provide the benefit of being cheaper to start or equip your workout.

This is because you can complete the exercise anywhere, anytime, with no need for weights (unless you are upping the intensity, it may seem easy but walk into this portion of isometric exercise). This is an awesome form of exercise for those people who have no time or are really trying to build strength in specific areas. Actually, this is an awesome way to supplement your six pack abs routine. Through the intensity of a harder isometric hold, you are going to be causing the six pack abs to go crazy!

How to Get Six Pack Abs with a Brown Paper Bag

Imagine this, what if a brown paper bags worked helped with getting a six pack. Want to know something? A brown paper bag is something to help with your six pack journey! Maybe not so much directly, as a cooler could help also, keep reading

Let's Look Into Developing A (Good) Habit!

Let's get back to our habit innate ability to form habits, but this is going to be a good one that is going to help us big time. So we are writing down and prioritizing our day, cool! A question could be raised on the idea of how a brown paper bag can help with getting your six pack and that is a fantastic question, here's the answer. It's a lunch bag (you couldn't tell the similarity with a cooler?!)

Priorities, especially for me came down to activities or tasks I needed to do that day. If you are anything like me, you will neglect to add sleep, meditation, and meal periods. When it came to those 3, I literally never had time. So do yourself a favor and write down brown paper bag on your daily priorities list.

So what are some things we should put into our brown paper bag to make lunch healthier? That is all dependent on if your brown paper bag can be chilled or refrigerated. Let's pretend you have regular access to refrigeration and how our brown paper bag can help with how to get six pack abs.

Leftovers are normally thrown out, and if you put an effort into creating a healthy meal the night before that's a waste!

Did you have chicken or ham last night? How about an oven roasted chicken, that's my favorite. What can we throw on that bad boy? Mayonnaise sounds good, NOT! What I would do is rip the chicken up and put it in a bag. Next I would take a whole grain or spinach wrap and fold it for later in a separate bag (makes it less soggy). Take a serving of hummus or an avocado slice and put them in a bag as well. Spinach, baby bok choy, or a green or red chard sounds good, how about some slender pepper rings? Put those together. Grab a plastic knife also. Read that again. You're getting protein, vitamins, a little bit of cards, some crunch and tons of flavor. You cut out the fat from mayo also. The ideas are really endless.

When you get on your lunch break all you have to do is unfold your wrap, lather the hummus on the bottom, place your veggies, then chicken and roll it up. You not only saved money and calories on an OTC lunch "hold me over", you're starting to create your own six pack abs diet!

How to get six pack abs with a brown paper bag should now be blatantly obvious. Not only are you staying away from fast food calories and fat, you're developing two great habits in one. Saving money with your own lunch as well as practicing healthy eating. What do you like to bring with you for lunch? Start writing down some ideas.

How To Get Six Pack Abs With A Pen and Paper!

We're going to hit off on a couple things while we continue our tweaks on how to get six pack abs! If you've been following this site for a while (good job if you have, shame – shame if you haven't!) you will have observed a couple of different things. One is I love analogies, LOVE THEM! Another thing you may have noticed is that I like to go over things a few times, and seeing the topic of six pack abs is so deep, we'll touch off on a few things, use a fast reiteration, and move on to today's topic!

Last time I posted on how to get those washboard abs I discussed the importance of thinking about breakfast before you started thinking about how stressful your day was going to be. I should add, if you stress easy and are often running late that by skipping the drive through or morning wait to give yourself junk should give you more time to get to work or school! Just saying.

The post before that discussed one of the most important things you can do in the morning in regards to getting those God like abs. Without going back to this post on how to get six pack abs, do you remember what it was and the stat I gave you? You're right, drinking water (nice, fresh, chilled) water – at least 16 ounces to be exact – will jump start your metabolism alone for around 90 minutes. Talk about getting free time! A jump started metabolism just by purifying yourself and quenching your thirst with nature's solvent!

How to get six pack abs by following instructions

Taking that you have drunk (or is it drank?) your 16 ounce glass of water already and eaten your breakfast, here's something you can do while you're chomping! Actually, once this becomes a habit of yours it will greatly assist you with attaining those defined abs.

Take a pen and paper, write a list of 1 through 10 on there. We are going to write not only the tasks needed with how to get a six pack, however also other things. 1 through 3 are the most pressing issues you need to get done, the other items are bonuses.

What is one thing you have to get done today? It would be nice to work on getting a six pack between work and dinner time, so throw that up there for number one. You just told yourself getting six pack abs, or at least working toward them, is your most important task of the day.

What are two other things that can dramatically improve your life today? Taking out the trash so you do not have to listen to your significant other complain is a good one. How about going to the hardware store and grabbing a power washer so you can nail the walls (outside of course) of your house?

In the end, once you place learning about how to get six pack abs, or working to attain them, at the top of your list the next job is to hold yourself accountable to doing the mandatory tasks involved! What a long sentence, that actually leads me to this point! If you can accomplish things, aside from feeling better about getting them done, you will also have created progression.

Constant progression leads to regular results. What that means at the end of the day is that your mission of getting six pack abs has become easier, and easier. Actually, in a few weeks you should begin seeing some results and start to believe that you are actually getting six pack abs!

So what does all this have to do with breakfast? Great question, I have found (although I have not seen a study on it yet, nor have I really searched to be honest) through my clients that reading or writing down tasks will make your meal period last a bit longer. What happens when it takes you longer to eat? You will become full at a much faster rate! You will slowly begin digesting instead of shoveling food down your throat to move on to the next thing. Aside from that, isn't planning when you can fit in the gym and figure out how to get six pack abs a bonus? I told ya so!

When discussing how to get six pack abs, one of the mandatory tasks is through exercise. Regardless if you consider them six pack exercises or simply as core strengthening exercises, ab training is a crucial foundation in regards to how to get six pack abs.

To the beginning ab enthusiast, abdominal exercises could be considered complete with only a few sit-ups. Aside from ending at a few crunches, some might try and over extend themselves during their exercise due to a lack of proper ab training and inexperience or simply doing the ab exercises incorrectly! Let's see how this post can help with how to get six pack abs!

How to Get Six Pack Abs Starting With the Basics

Six pack abs have been a hot topic for ages, this should implicitly imply to you they are not new. One of the best exercises, and more dangerous I should add, however lost a lot of popularity after providing so many results for decades prior. Can you guess which one it is? Read on and you'll see if you were correct!

Building a Case For The Sit-Up

Sit-ups are looked down upon by some, they can be an easy starting point on your quest for six pack abs. Actually, often when I am asked by clients which exercises are most effective or that they should have as a staple in that quest I ask them specifically about sit-ups. I normally get the confused puppy look (imagine a puppy confused, looking at you tilted with one ear raised). In regards to core strength I don't know a better exercise that works as powerfully at developing total core strength.

A properly done sit-up induces force and works not just the ab section, however the lower back as well. The problem with sit-ups is that they have the unfriendly ability to cause injury or even unneeded muscle soreness more commonly than most other six pack exercises. Make sure you do them properly and after a few weeks you'll love the results.

Commercial Time Is A Great Time To Freeze

An exercise group I like to do during commercial breaks on TV are planks. Every form of a properly done plank or "bridge" as some like to call the group can target various segments of different muscle groups.

Something I really try to focus on when doing planks is to ensure a prolonged and solid contraction through each rep. This exercise is also enjoyable for my babies; sometimes on a rainy day they will ask if we can do some planks (of course we turn it into a game).

As this six pack exercise has a vastly lower chance of causing injury I have zero issue with them doing them. What decent parent would pass up the opportunity to encourage regular exercise in their children?! Actually, although this post is geared more toward specific, basic, exercises how to get six pack abs is easiest to be accomplished when encouraged at an early age. That's a point worth adding in, I digress so we move on.

How to get six pack abs with Super Man?!

Another exercise that I find helps with how to get six pack abs is named after a super hero, can you guess which one? Here's a hint, he's the guy with the red cape and super tight clothes. The "superman" really helps target the muscles responsible for your core and really helps with working your core. Not so much your abs, however it really hits the small of your back, unless you take my holding the contraction trick for your abs mentioned in the previous exercise - then it's a core workout! If you can envision Super Man flying, you can do this exercise, and I'll explain it as it is not so main stream as other exercises are.

You lay on your stomach, face down. Extend your arms out and point your thumbs toward the sky. Next, point your toes inward as if you are trying to touch your knees or your shins with them. Like other core exercises you also want to contract your abs. Lift your arms up slightly, with your thumbs remaining pointed toward the sky and lift your legs with your toes pointed in. While you have your abs contracted, you now want to lower your shoulder blades pulled down toward the middle of your back.

There's a pretty good starting point for you if I do say so myself. These exercises are an easy way to help you get started with your quest to six pack abs!

We Need Hydration, ever Consider Alkaline Water?

Fast riddle for you, can you tell me the correlation between six pack abs and an overheated car in the desert? Any clue? I asked a few clients and I had answers that contained cactus' (not so incorrect, although I couldn't figure what they had to do with *how to get six pack abs*), oasis's, and mirages. I was a little nervous when one of my clients said how to get six pack abs and the car overheating in the dessert were mirages. They politely informed me I was doing an awesome job either way and it was just the first thing they had come to mind.

So what do they have in common? How to get six pack abs is a partial sentence with nouns, adjectives, verbs, and so on. A dried up river and an overheated car are both nouns with an adjective in front of them, but it has nothing to do with sentence structure.

How about a lack of water?

A dried up river could lead directly into a desert where there's an overheated car. And as far as how to get six pack abs water plays a critical element in your quest for the perfect set of washboard abs! Want to know why? Take a guess (I have been in a pain in the butt mood all day for some reason).
Granted alkaline water will decrease the acid levels in your but that is actually not what I am looking for answer-wise.

It does in some sense actually have to do with what happens when salt meets alkaline water in the body and helps trigger the electro responses we need for life. But that isn't what I am getting at between the car, desert, and how to get six pack abs.

Actually, the answer is not so much water, nor alkaline water, however the tremendous need for it and lack thereof in all three components of my riddle. Actually I am going to take it a step further and tell you when your body needs water the most! If you guessed after a run, jog, or long exercise routine, you are right that you do need hydration.

However that is not when your body needs it the most. Actually, when you feed water to your body in its highest time of need, you could potentially spike your metabolism by as much as 24 percent for up to 90 minutes. That is, of course, if you drink 16 ounces of chilled water! Alright, I'll tell you when that opportune time is, it's when you wake up.

Got a theory on how that works in regards to how to get six pack abs?

Why does water first thing in the morning help with getting six pack abs so efficiently? Picture this and it should make more sense to you. Do you sleep the way you are supposed to, you know the full 8 hour shebang? What happens if you breathe with your mouth? You have eight hours of dehydration (not to mention some really kicking breath). Aside from quenching your thirst, you sort of "startle" your metabolism into moving its fat consuming butt!

<u>Do You Start Off With Stress?</u>

Speaking of starting off, what about the effect your first waking thoughts have on your journey of how to get six pack abs? Do you know how your thoughts influence your journey first thing in the morning? Most people start by sleeping in and then waking up wondering where they're going to stop for breakfast. That is, especially now a day, when your stress level starts to consume you (of course, only if you let it.

So where what am I going to go with? I am not saying you should start doing crunches or sit-ups in bed. I am not even saying to tell yourself you HAVE to work out later on. Actually, it is a task that many people outsource in the morning. It's called Dunkin Donuts or McDonalds serving you a fast quick fix because you stayed in bed dwelling on your day instead of how you're going to fill your body with nutrients.

Money is also stressful, so I thought about how you can save money while on your journey of how to get six pack abs. It happened as I was driving by Dunkin Donuts while I was thinking about it and almost went off the road. I also realized that I get far too excited far too easily. I actually remember what happened, I started swerving as soon as I said "that's not *how to get six pack abs*" and I had my first A HA moment of the day.

Instead of wasting money on yummy commercials and processed garbage, wake up a few moments earlier and make something healthy. If you need more beauty sleep you can just as easily prepare it the night before!

Want some suggestions?

What about organic chicken sausage made by Al Fresco? Protein and some fat are there (it's morning, you want stuff to burn right?). Take that a small step further and couple that up with some filling fiber and maybe a Greek Yogurt. Or you could take some greens, juice them, and throw them in with Greek yogurt and make a healthy smoothie?

I am guilt of being a breakfast boycotter....

Breakfast was always my downfall. I benched 300 pounds regularly in high school, I ran, I consumed tons of protein, and I still didn't have six pack abs. I was not a breakfast eater so my metabolism acted like a car that has 200,000 miles, it started really slow (plus I drank hot tea or coffee instead of chilled water).

Want another way eating breakfast will help with your journey on getting that six pack? Look at this math: people who skip breakfast are 4.5 times more likely to suffer from bulging belly syndrome!

So we've cut out spending money and nailed that stressor, we've seen a scary stat on skipping breakfast, and you have an amazing breakfast that's fast and delicious!

It's Not The End....

You've made it to the end of this book, congratulations! I want you to realize, this is not the end, and actually this is only the beginning. This is the beginning of your new life and your walk toward body transformation. Don't not fear it, embrace it.

www.ingramcontent.com/pod-product-compliance
Lightning Source LLC
Chambersburg PA
CBHW070546010626
45795CB00016BC/914